50 Things You Can Do Today to Beat Depression

50 Things You Can Do Today to Beat Depression
Copyright © Paul Vincent 2005

ISBN   1-84426-337-1

First Published 2005 by
UPFRONT PUBLISHING LTD
Cambridgeshire

Printed by Copytech UK Ltd

50 Things You Can Do Today to Beat Depression

Paul Vincent

This book is designed to be short and to the point. As the title suggests, it contains fifty ways you can beat depression today. It also contains far more. In fact, it is my belief that if you give this book an honest hour of your time, you can and will cure your depression for good. All you have to say is, 'What the hell, I'll give it a chance,' and follow the instructions as you go along.

You will need:

- An hour on your own.
- A pen.
- About fifteen pieces of blank paper.
- A clean empty litter bin (a cardboard box will do).
- A clock or watch.
- A mirror that is big enough to see your whole face.
- The TV definitely off, but perhaps a CD player or iPod to hand, but turned off at this stage.

No alcohol. This is not going to work if you're plastered.

Oh and here's a warning:

If you are allergic to nuts, don't eat nuts.

What do I mean? I cannot possibly know all about your life and your health, so when you follow any advice it is your responsibility to do so sensibly.

Finally, before we get stuck in: 'depression' is an overused word which has come to encompass countless problems and symptoms ranging from everything from anxiety to insomnia. Accordingly, I will use the word quite loosely throughout or often I will just say 'illness' and let's assume it is usually shorthand for 'the problems we are facing' whatever those may be.

Here goes...

Depression is the single most prevalent illness in Western society. Why is this?

Among other reasons, it's because depression drains people of energy. It drains people of energy, self confidence and hope. In other words, the illness itself robs you of the very qualities you would need to cure it.

Think about it. An illness that by its very nature stops you from curing it. It stops you from *believing* it can be cured; it stops you having the *strength* to cure it; often it stops people from even having strong desires, so it stops you even *desiring* to cure it.

How clever is that?

It is genius.

If you were an evil scientist trying to mess with people's minds, you would be hard pressed to think up something cleverer than depression. It's such a successful illness that the cost in the UK alone of the medication, counselling, lost work and ancillary illnesses is thought to be over £3 billion a year. Severe depression is thought to affect up to 10% of the population at any one time, and over a lifetime, *most* people will have suffered from it at some stage. And yet despite this extraordinary cost and the number of people fighting it every day, there seems to be no end in sight. Now that is a successful illness.

I will make no apology for stressing this concept again and again. Depression is so successful because it robs you of the means and desire to cure it. Oh okay. It *almost* robs you: after all you've taken the trouble to buy this book, haven't you? It hasn't won the battle just yet.

So, what can we do?

Firstly let's get the concept fixed firmly in our heads that the brain is an organ like any other body organ. It can need rest, it can get damaged, it can be strong, and it can get an illness. In this instance, your brain has managed to get itself an illness and this illness is inflicting on you some of the following:

- Tiredness.
- Lack of confidence.
- Dankness.
- Inability to sleep.
- A need to sleep too much.
- A need to eat too much or too little.
- Lack of energy.
- 'Hyper' patches.
- Despondency.
- Selfishness.
- Introspection.
- Drinking.
- Gambling.
- Not able to get out enough.
- Not able to enjoy life.
- A need to spend too much money.
- Inability to concentrate.
- Inability to be a good friend.

...and that list is probably just scraping the surface.

So this is the first key concept I want to press home:

Your brain has an illness and it is inflicting symptoms on you. Like any organ or muscle in the body, it will respond to exercise, medications, good nutrition and generally being treated well.

Note that there is nothing contentious or revolutionary about this concept. I'm not trying to be contentious or revolutionary: I simply want to explain how we can become happy for the rest of our lives. To recap therefore:

Depression is a work of genius. It robs you of the very energy and hope that you need to cure it.

Your brain has an illness and it is inflicting symptoms on you. Like any organ or muscle in the body, it will respond to exercise, medications, good nutrition and generally being treated well.

So...

Read the next sentence very carefully.

DEPRESSION IS AN ILLNESS THAT ROBS PEOPLE OF THE BELIEF THAT THEY CAN CURE IT.

Right. Now cover that sentence with your hand and see if you can still remember it clearly.

I am assuming that 90% of people just covered that sentence up and repeated it. If you didn't, is it because you have decided upfront to skimp your way through this book? Why? It's only short, and we've barely begun. Or is it because you don't believe this cure is going to work? Why do you believe that? Because your brain has an illness that is robbing you of the belief that cures can work? Or is it because you think I am talking rubbish? In which case, hell, you didn't give me a very long honeymoon period.

Nag nag nag.

You will find I will nag occasionally. It doesn't worry me if you end up not liking me; it *does* worry me if we don't take this chance to cure you.

What did Nike, the Greek god of trainers say? Just do it.

One more time then, and we can move on. Everyone please read the last sentence that is in capitals again and then put your hand over the page to see if you can remember it.

Now sit up in your chair and clap your hands twice, loudly. Why? Because depression robs people of energy.

And you are going to need to progressively raise your metabolism to fight back. By this I mean raise both your body's metabolism and the metabolism of your brain. Clap your hands twice again, louder. You did clap your hands, yes? Because I promise you this book will work, but you actually have to do everything I suggest.

There is no doubt a very small percentage of people reading this who still feel they were too cool or important to clap their hands. Consider this...

You have a friend who has a terrible headache. He or she is holding a packet of headache tablets and reading the instructions on the back. Four hours later you ask them how it's going, but you discover they are still standing there reading the back of the packet.

'Oh I'm not going to take the tablets,' they say. 'It's enough just to read the packet.'

What do you think of your friend? At what point did you start laughing at them?

Sit up in your chair again and clap your hands again, twice, loudly.

Ah, me; my favourite subject.

I suffered from depression all my adult life; from about the age of 14 until about 40. I think what annoys me most looking back was the sheer waste of time it involved. I should have been out there enjoying myself and instead I was sapped of energy and so often let life pass me by. I think I missed out on really enjoying my children's early years and... oh I won't go on; it's too depressing.

I tried 'everything': tablets, counselling, self-help books, exercise: you name it. And do you know what? They all helped... a bit. So don't let me put you off pursuing any of these avenues. But during that period I became convinced of one important thing. I am so convinced that this particular concept is crucial that it is the next sentence I want us to learn. Yes I know it's mildly irritating, and I promise the whole book is not like this, but I want you to read carefully:

NO **ONE** CURE WILL CHANGE MY LIFE 100%.

Place your hand over the sentence and check that you can remember it.

Why would it? If you had flu you might take tablets, go to bed and take lots of fluids. If you decide you are prone to flu, you might consider having a flu vaccine the following year. So that's at least four measures you would instinctively take. If you broke an arm you would have the bone set, then have a cast made, then take pain killers and then you'd rest the arm for several weeks. Again, that's four measures. The brain is far more intricate than a broken bone, and when you bear in mind the long list of symptoms a couple of pages earlier, depression is surprisingly complicated. So why would only one cure be the total solution?

Sit up again and clap your hands twice, loudly. Now read carefully again:

DEPRESSION IS AN ILLNESS THAT ROBS PEOPLE OF THE BELIEF THAT THEY CAN CURE IT.

and

NO **ONE** CURE WILL CHANGE MY LIFE 100%.

So?

So, as promised I am now going to suggest **fifty** ways you can improve your life **2% or more.** And what's more, it's going to change your life.

Over the last few years I set up a number of websites; they were all on the subject of depression but each of them had slightly different slants. I listed the measures that had helped me personally to get over depression and I also listed the most common solutions that mainstream professionals offer which I had either never tried, or which hadn't worked for me personally. On the sites, I stressed that although I am medically trained, I have had no lengthy training in psychiatry: I am essentially a member of the public whose life has been ruled by depression.

I had a simple mission. Of the ideas suggested, I wanted people to tell me what they found worked best, and how. I wanted to know of any drawbacks and, well, *all* information and bright ideas were welcome. I particularly wanted people to tell me of other remedies not on the list they had tried over the years. I then posted the best of these ideas and I asked people to try any of them they fancied and tell me about their experiences.

After a number of months I was able to hone the websites down to solutions that had very high success rates and I then 'experimented' by suggesting different orders in which people could try them, and I experimented with my tone: trying everything from the 'Oh poor you' approach to the hectoring of a sergeant major. A massive 210,000 people have now used the websites and I am constantly overwhelmed by how pleasant and helpful everyone is and was. From LA to India, from Reykjavik to Melbourne, I got hour after hour of emails to read every single day offering insights and sharing experiences. It was fascinating and moving; exhilarating, exhausting, and deeply life affirming. It was by far and away the best thing I have ever done in my life. What did I end up with? Well a huge bag of solutions from Cognitive Therapy style ideas to putting nutmeg in coffee: and from these I have taken the cream of the crop.

About once a day I would get an email where the sole motivation of the writer appeared to be the need to be rude to me – particularly during my sergeant major phase. A common one would be something like, 'I can see how this might work for people with mild depression, but you've obviously never had real depression mate, otherwise you wouldn't have the temerity to make some of these suggestions.' They would then start swearing at me. Perversely these same people would also tend to ask me what the 'answer' was. So although they believed they had a worse case of depression than other people, they also believed that they would only need one 'cure.' To go back to the analogy of a broken arm: if it had multiple breakages instead of one then you would expect the treatment to be more convoluted, not less: you certainly wouldn't expect there to be one sole cure. As for whether I had 'real' depression...

I had 'real' depression. For example, there was the year where I could no longer speak. I am quite a chatty person, but one summer I discovered that I would get about two or three words into a sentence and my brain simply wouldn't let me continue. So I would start the sentence again but then I would have even less success. People either looked at me wide eyed and backed slowly out of the room or, more interestingly, they thought I was being bad mannered and rude. Then there was the time when I discovered I could no longer read. Judging by my post bag this is a surprisingly common symptom. I could just about read the headlines of newspapers, but no more than that. I could look at the pictures in magazines, but I couldn't read the captions. It was bit of handicap, as I had a paying hobby at the time reviewing books. Then there were the anxiety attacks where I kept vomiting. I am quite strong willed and promised myself not to go below a certain weight, but it's a little hard if your food won't stay down.

I could bore you with more details, and I am sure there are lots of people around the world with worse problems than me, but by the end of this book you can accuse me of anything you like, but I won't allow the idea that I don't know what it is to be depressed or anxious.

Another common email I get is along the lines of, 'My doctor said I should get more exercise. How is that going to solve all my problems?'

I can answer that very easily. It's not.

Exercise is the third most common suggestion that doctors make to depressed patients. It is a truly excellent idea, and we will cover it later in the book. But no, it won't solve all your problems. I look at it this way: at each and every juncture we have to ask ourselves a remarkably simple question. What will make our lives a notional 2% better? In the case of exercise; getting the heart pumping and getting fit and active would definitely make us at least 2% better compared to sitting in a chair waiting for a cure for depression to drop through the ceiling.

The thing to grasp again and again is the '2%' concept. What exactly is our excuse for *not* getting some exercise?

The biggest surprise I got from my postbag was the reaction from the medical fraternity. I was expecting trouble. Who was this upstart treading in the venerable field of psychology without so much as a by your leave or a framed certificate on the wall? I needn't have worried. Every single medically qualified person who contacted me was helpful and pleasant. One Professor of psychiatry in America even wrote to apologise to me. 'I am terribly sorry, but in our clinic we have copied your website and we give it out as a hand out to our patients. Is that okay?' Of course it's okay.

To my amazement this happened again and again. Clinic after clinic around the world had started using my suggestions and solutions as hand outs. I was totally stunned... and pleased, of course. One clinician even wrote me a lovely letter saying, 'I myself have taken your advice, and it has brought so much joy to my life and that of my husband.'

I contacted a number of councillors and psychiatrists for advice when writing this book and I am indebted to all of them. In an idle moment I asked one of them why I had been given such a warm reception. She didn't have to think about her answer. She said, 'In your position, you can say a lot of things we professionals would like to say but feel we can't. You are allowed to nag and laugh and cherry pick from different disciplines. You are allowed to suggest word of mouth remedies with as much enthusiasm as when you delve into pure science. You're not anti-doctors and you're not anti-homespun cures. In short, you tell it like it is.'

Stand up.

Have your mirror in front of you so that you can see your face.

Now say out loud all the recent problems you have had and all the things that have been annoying you or getting you down. Take as long as you like, but throughout you must watch your own lips as you say the words. You must feel those words leave your body, as easily as the air leaves your lungs.

Now pause for breath a moment and think of an entirely different type of problem that you have been dwelling on, then in your own time start the exercise again.

When you start to feel foolish about some of the problems you are coming out with, you may stop, provided you have done the exercise for a good minute in total and you watched your lips for the whole time.

Now consider the last problem you mentioned out loud.

Get a piece of paper from your pile and place it on your lap or table in front of you.

Now stare at it. Imagine a visual scene on that piece of paper that represents the problem. Perhaps it is the people involved in this problem or, say, your boss at work. Can you see them clearly on the paper?

Now imagine that scene shrinking on the paper: shrinking like a photocopier shrinks an image. Shrink it smaller and smaller until it is half the size it was before.

Then shrink it again to half of that size, and then half again, and as you do so drain all the colour out of it. Drain all the life out of it.

Can you still see it? Can you see how it is diminished and dulled and rendered lifeless?

Now fold the edges of the paper up and over so that the 'image' is covered.

Now crumple up the paper.

Get the paper in both hands and scrunch it up. Really put some effort in; scrunch it up good and proper. Now throw it in the bin. Have a look at it in the bin. That's where it's staying.

Now that you've got the hang of that, repeat the exercise for the first problem you spoke out loud.

It feels good doesn't it?

One piece of research shows that when a woman is 'down' she will put on cheerful music or perhaps spend the evening pampering herself. Wonderful. The same research showed that men tend to put on gloomy music (a nice bit of Joy Division, Tom Waits or some group where the multi-millionaire lead singer killed himself after a lengthy drugs problem) and they will drink.

Lads oh lads oh lads. You can't beat depression with depression. So please, if possible, now spend a minute rigging up a bit of music; something you really like, obviously, but something upbeat; something, perhaps that you associate with happy experiences in your life. Have it on in the background but not too loud. If you don't like music, then fair enough, give that a miss.

Now read this list of words out loud:

- GLITTER.
- SHINING.
- HAPPY.
- SUNSHINE.
- RICH.
- GOOD.
- SENSATIONAL.
- EXCITEMENT.
- ELECTRICITY.
- TREAT.
- GOODIES.
- SUCCESS.

- HAPPINESS.
- LAUGHTER.
- PASSION.
- FRESH.
- FRUITFUL.
- SMILE.

Read it again out loud, but with two differences; this time keep a big smile on your face throughout and open your eyes wider so that they twinkle, and with each word (while smiling) over-enunciate every syllable. e.g. Sensational is: SEN- SAY – SHUN – ALL

Your voice sounds seductive, sensuous and very good.

There are several independent pieces of research that show that just saying positive words makes you feel good. Like all the suggestions in this book: it's free and it's proven, and you can do them over and over again. What's more, each time you do them they work even better. Free, easy and effective. It doesn't get better than that.

While we are delving into science here is another interesting finding:

In the 90s there was some research where they got students to keep diaries over the course of a year. Half of them had to spend thirty minutes a day reading last year's diary, and the other students had to spend the same amount of time planning future activities. Guess who were happier? The people who made plans were happier. Far far happier. The people who were forced to dwell on the past became more depressed. Depression itself has a tendency to make you dwell on the past. It's a vicious circle.

So:

Get a piece of paper and spend the next few minutes choosing a list of five things you want to do in the next twelve months. Stick to goals that are possible, please: 'Marry George Clooney/Angelina Jolie' is not an option.

Review the list and check you like it. If need be start again on a new piece of paper. The list should end up being clear and concise and there should be nothing else on the page.

Now fold up the piece of paper neatly and place it in your bag or briefcase.

You must carry this with you wherever you go in the next year.

Turn a piece of paper sideways on and draw six large circles that don't interlock.

Now turn them into faces; three male, three female. Give them hair, noses, ears, hats, scarves, little bodies... anything you like really. The only rule is that they should all be smiling. Big broad smiles. Giggly smiles. Cheeky smiles. Anything you like, so long as all the smiles are different.

A piece of research published last year showed that the five biggest problems in relationships were in the following fields:

- People need time together.

- People need some sort of joint activity or interest they can share.

- People need to feel they are 'heard'

- People need to feel they can express their identity.

- People need to feel that their grievances are addressed, not ignored.

Get a new piece of paper and choose one relationship important to you: partner, friend, child, parent or indeed anyone you spend a lot of time with. It could even be someone who now lives a distance away and who you mostly contact by phone.

Now write down some ideas about how some of these concepts could be gently used by you to improve the life quality of the OTHER person. How might they be able to express their identity more? Are they getting a chance to be heard? Have their grievances been addressed or just buried? Perhaps, and more importantly, you want to find time to let them show you all about their favourite hobby, or perhaps get them chatting a bit about their plans for the future.

This tip may take a little thought and time, so give yourself a couple of minutes. It works surprisingly well.

Of the thousands of emails I have received, I had countless from people who gave this tip a lot of thought and found it worked wonders. I had just the one email from someone who said, 'I can't see how this helps *me*.' It reminded me of the story Barry Humphries tells in his book *More Please*. When he finally gave up the booze he realised he had previously devoted the majority of his waking hours to his alcoholism.

He said to his doctor, 'How can I fill my time?'

The doctor replied, 'Have you ever considered helping other people?'

Barry Humphries self-deprecatingly admits that was the most revolutionary thing he had ever heard.

What are your core strengths?

If you love your own company should you become a teacher or a lighthouse keeper? If you are flamboyant should you work on the stage or in a library? It's obvious isn't it?

I am very keen in this book to keep the concepts clear and concise; so much so that I will run the risk of being seen to state the obvious. I feel that too often people over complicate what they have to say just to try and 'prove' they are an expert and you are not.

So again I don't apologise for stating a key concept that's very important, but also very obvious:

Usually, in life, it's best to play to your strengths.

In the US at the moment there is some excellent work being done in this field. It can be very loosely summarized by saying that there are three big elements to happiness:

1   Reduce your anxieties, such as how you can pay the mortgage, pass an exam etc.

2   Have some elements in your weekly regime that you enjoy: after all if your week includes nothing that you like, that is obviously worth addressing.

3   Play to your strengths.

On the next three pages we will look at these three elements.

I can't pay your mortgage for you, or finish your college assignment but I can suggest the following. It is very effective.

Get a piece of paper, and on the left hand side write a column of all the practical problems you have, leaving a bit of a space between each. Include the tiny stuff, like 'Must finish an essay' to the really big stuff like 'Sort out credit card debts.'

On the right hand side now write the possible solutions. These might be things like 'Pick up phone and make appointment to talk to the bank,' or 'Pick up phone and chat to that friend I had a misunderstanding with.'

I'm sure you've got the hang of that and what you need to do, so I won't waste anyone's time by labouring this one, but do spend a decent amount of time doing a proper job of this task: it is very important.

Shut your eyes and visualise your week. Monday, Tuesday... through to Saturday and Sunday. What are your favourite parts? Really take your time to visualise each day in turn. Is a favourite bit putting your feet up on Friday? Seeing a movie with friends? Saturday morning sport in the park, or at a tennis club? A DVD and a box of chocolates? A pub quiz? Walking the dog?

Now plan how you can do a bit more of these activities:

Firstly, clear your mind and now spend thirty seconds to a minute working out if it is possible, hypothetically, to set up a more regular time to pursue certain hobbies or see certain people.

Now clear your mind again and spend a minute having a think to see if you can't branch out your interests a bit or introduce some slight variations on something that is getting stale.

Now spend a minute running through in your mind some fun things you used to do in the past. Can you resurrect a pleasure that has somehow dropped out of your roster? Or alternatively, as I said previously, could you take on board what a friend or partner would like to do?

If you have young children a really great idea that we found a complete godsend was to book the same sitter for the same three hours every single week. The teenager was very happy to do it because it represented a regular income and we didn't have to keep ringing round just for the honour of leaving the house together once a week.

Our sitter was so keen to 'keep her job' she even used to send her sister in her place when she was busy. Or you might have a relative who can sit for you or there might be a babysitting circle in your area; it would certainly be cheaper. With our three hours a week we would see the latest film or go out for a drink or try a new eatery that had opened in town. If you're on a tight budget you'll find some alternative bright ideas later in this book.

A lot of people feel guilty for enjoying themselves. They see that they are using up household resources, such as time and money, for their selfish own pleasure. Don't feel guilty, just do it, within reason obviously. Our big battle at the moment is with depression: if it involves a few extra treats to get that notional 2% advantage then, I'd say that's pretty fair.

Sometimes every day phrases show a lot of wisdom, and phrases like 'take him out of himself' or 'that really got her out of herself' are surprisingly profound. We all know what it means and it's a good thing. We should all do it more often and help others to do it too.

So to focus further on this line of thought; can you think of a specific treat you can plan in the next few days that will play to your strengths and lead to some enjoyment? I would suggest a 'doing' activity would be best, by which I mean entertainment such as seeing a film, or a sport such as playing squash, pool, or seeing a game rather than, say, sitting having a 'quiet drink' which, let's face it, can be code for 'a chance to dwell on your problems.'

Now visualise the activity you have just planned. Have an indulgent twenty seconds dwelling on the precise details of it, working out how to make it happen and imagining actually doing it.

Make yourself a promise now to actually carry out the treat you have just envisaged. Don't forget that depression is always waiting for a moment to assert itself; between now and the time of your proposed treat, it may try and 'talk you out of it' it might say 'Oh what's the point?' or 'Oh I'm not in the mood now.' If you don't carry out your treat then depression wins. Yet again.

Spend a few moments considering your core strengths. This list may give you some ideas, but it is by no means an exhaustive list of positive human traits:

- I love exploring.
- I am a loving person.
- I am inquisitive.
- I am spiritual.
- I am a nurturer or carer.
- I am energetic.
- I am thoughtful.
- I am a career person.
- I am a people person.
- I am an organiser.
- I am a team person.
- I am a calming influence.
- I am dynamic.
- I entertain.
- I am a broker.
- I am a busy person.
- I am creative.
- I am careful.
- I persevere.
- I am a teacher.

Pick three or four concepts that sum you up – they don't have to be on the list above and more than four is fine.

Now pick an extra one that is something positive people might say about you behind your back.

Put them all down on a piece of paper, because we are getting back to them later. In the meantime though, spend a minute considering your home life and your work life. Are there any ways you can tweak your current life so that you can play to your strengths better? Would it be possible to delegate any jobs which are not your forte and perhaps take a stronger role in areas where you are more gifted? If you are considering careers or a career change, a lot of career books, such as the Which Guide to Choosing a Career will stress the personal qualities you would need for different jobs. It may be worth looking into something like that in the coming weeks, even if you are not looking for change, then you may want to see what they say about the job you are currently in and consider if you need to change any of your skills or perspectives.

Some of the ideas I suggest in this book are about setting up a chain of positive events for your future well being, and here is the first of them.

A number of people sent this idea in to me from different parts of the world, and it is so simple and yet so effective that it deserves a fanfare of some sort before I unveil its quiet genius.

Start a diary.

Yes, I know I said earlier that reading a diary can be a downer, but this is a diary with a difference.

Every day in a diary you must write down one positive thing that has happened. It could be a joke that made you smile, or a new series of your favourite programme starting on TV. It could be something kind you did for someone, a little anecdote from work, a good mark from school, something beautiful you saw on the way home that day, or something funny a pet did.

Do it every single day and never allow yourself to write anything negative or neutral. Be happy to include really tiny stuff; it's very healthy to appreciate the smaller joys of life and not just the bigger achievements.

In the months ahead if you ever feel low, get your diary out and read a few pages. Our lives often prove to be more varied, remarkable, fun and enriching than we credit. Every single person who contacted me about this tip gave it full marks.

COGNITIVE – From the word 'Cognition' – 'the mental act or process by which knowledge is acquired.'

Go back to Chapter Four entitled 'Sen-say-shun-all' and put a huge smile on your face, open your eyes wide and make them twinkle, then read out loud the positive word list again.

Now let's have a little delve into the area of cognitive therapy...

Get a clean piece of paper.

1 Identify a flash point in your life: an event that made you depressed or lose your temper perhaps. Write down a description of the actual event. e.g 'my boss shouted at me.'

2 Now write down the effect it had on you, e.g. 'depressed', 'anxious', 'it made me hyperventilate' or whatever. Now give each of these words a rating 0-100% for the severity of the symptom. e.g. anxious 80% angry 95% or helpless 70%.

3 Now write down what was going through your mind just BEFORE you started to feel this way. If there were any other thoughts at all, then just list them, preferably as a short sentence. Any visual images? Any childhood flashbacks? Now look at the list and circle the thought that seems most important. e.g 'I suck at my job' or 'I am such a loser'.

4 Write down some evidence that supports this proposition.

5   Now on a fresh sheet of paper, write down all the evidence from your entire life that does NOT support this proposition. Take your time. 'My previous boss praised me.' 'A customer told me last week how helpful I was.' 'I got a pay rise last year.' 'At least half my colleagues are far worse than me.' 'It's a pretty hard job, so of course I make mistakes.' 'I make far fewer mistakes than when I started.' 'If they replaced me they would need one and half people in my place to do as much as I do.' You might add to this list by thinking of what a good friend would say to you. It could be a best friend from the past or even an 'ideal' friend. What positive things might they point out?

6   Read the 'positive' piece of paper again and finally look at your list of words in section two and rate how you now feel about them. e.g. Depressed 30%.

7   Get this 'negative' piece of paper and place it face down underneath your pile of clean paper.

8   Now leave the 'positive' list out in plain view.

There is classic piece of recent research that shows that gardeners and hairdressers are happier than most, and what's more the same research identified why.

Apparently we humans enjoy smallish tasks where we can set a goal e.g. digging a border and planting some flower seeds, or making a mop of hair look more stylish. The task has a result we can see: a weeded flower bed on day one and, in the future, we see the flowers come up. The task also has the advantage of being achievable.

Compare this to suddenly deciding to write a novel. Writing a novel is no doubt laudable but you are not going to see a result for a very long time and as a first timer you are unlikely to get published. To add insult to injury, there will probably be some newspaper story about a first time novelist who got paid a huge advance and who then sold thousands of books, and this will make us feel inadequate because our half written book is just sitting unsold on a shelf gathering dust.

So. Have a little think about one of your favourite pastimes: an interest or hobby that lends itself to breaking down into smallish parcels with identifiable goals. This is likely to be one of the ideas you considered a few pages ago. See if you can rethink it slightly so that you can parcel it up into bite sized achievements you can go for in the coming weeks.

You may want to plan specifically when in the next fortnight you will be pursuing that pastime and how.

17 TIME TO SIT UP STRAIGHT AGAIN

Sit up straight, please.

Think of an instance in your life where you have been happy or successful. An incident where you have been the person you want to be. Perhaps helping a customer, or making a deal, or a time you were on a successful date or shining in a stage play or... well, it's up to you.

Hold your hands on your lap with your fingers interlocked. Shut your eyes and imagine all the details of this successful situation. See all the details in the room or in the background; imagine them clearly one by one; see them brightly. See clearly how you look in that situation. See how you stand and how you smile and talk.

This is the real you.

Feel yourself breathing in and out over and over again, slowly and resolutely. Feel your fingers interlocked and squeeze them together a few times.

Practice this, perhaps using a different positive memory. Or perhaps just imagine how you would like to be, how you would like to deal with people and situations. What the hell, imagine yourself in the car of your dreams or the house of your dreams, or on a dream holiday, or any other situation that you would associate with bliss. You can do this all day long for all it matters, but certainly spend a full minute doing it now. No skimping please.

Depression can strike without warning or conversely it can be as predictably regular as the sunrise. A very famous pop singer once said, 'I'm depressed every morning. So first thing, I leave my apartment in New York and I have a brisk walk around the block, buy a paper and coffee. That usually breaks the back of it.'

Happily, by contrast, a good mood can also come seemingly from nowhere. Someone might remark, 'You're in a good mood today' or 'It's nice to see someone so happy.' It's often only when you hear that that you realise what a good mood you're in. Or it's sometimes not until you're in a good mood that you realise how depressed you've been in recent weeks. I mention this because I think it is important to recognise that no matter how effective a cure is, there will always be peaks and troughs and it can be very hard to get a true sense of whether you are winning the battle against depression or not. In fact, because of this, most authorities won't 'allow' anyone to consider themselves depressed unless the symptoms have prevailed for more than two weeks.

With that in mind, I would suggest that for the next few weeks you refrain from taking stock of how good or bad you feel, except on the odd occasion during the next hour, when I say so. Firstly, a snapshot will tell you little or nothing, and secondly I think it's counter productive.

To draw a parallel: we have all had friends who try to give up smoking. When we observe them, we can usually tell which of them will succeed and which will fail. For example, the friends who keep telling us exactly how long it is since they last had a cigarette, usually fail.

'It's been two days, three hours and eleven seconds since my last cigarette,' you hear them say. Why do people like that fail? Because they are filling their every waking thought with an obsession about smoking: they are telling their brain that smoking is the most important thing to them. Similarly, when people are on a diet, the ones who do worst are the ones who give us a blow by blow account of how it's going: they are obsessing all day about… food.

I may not know much, but I know this for sure; the one thing a depressive cannot afford to obsess about is depression. It would be like saying, 'My trouble is I dwell on my problems all day: problems such as…' and then start listing those very problems.

I've particularly noticed that when some people take anti-depressant medication they give a blow by blow account along the lines of 'It's not working yet, it's not working yet…' These same people a few months later say, 'Oh I've just come off the tablets so I'm low at the moment.' They can't have it both ways. If they took the time they've spent dwelling on their symptoms and used it to throw themselves into ancillary remedies and cures, they would probably see better results.

Now I've got that off my chest, let's crack on with the next exercise…

Whenever something vexes you, or you find you are feeling negative about yourself, then do the following.

Imagine someone who is a good friend to you. It could be an 'ideal' friend or it could be a parent, an old school friend or a partner. It doesn't matter. What would they say to you about the subject that is annoying you? You might even be able to remember specific advice that they have given you in the past, and adapt that.

Sometimes we keep our problems to ourselves and in fact if we told a partner or friend about a problem they would offer great advice. The reason we don't tell them about the problem might be because we don't like to trouble them, or we like to look strong or the more we talk the more we feel a bit foolish about worrying about such a small problem.

Have a little think about whether you might like to chat to someone you know about a problem. But in the meantime, *imagine* what they would say to you. In your view is it good advice? Then act on it.

20 AN EXERCISE INVOLVING EXERCISE

If an athlete goes for a practice run and pushes themselves to get a slightly better time; they may or not succeed. As they place their hands on their hips and stand trying to get their breath back what, in your opinion, is the chance of them being depressed at that exact moment? About zero.

We all know that exercise releases hormones that make us feel good; in fact, most research shows it is more effective than medication, curing up to 60% more people permanently. Another piece of research showed that depressed people spent an average of two extra hours sitting down per day compared to people who were happy. It's common sense really. What is less widely known is that the more often you take exercise, the better the body gets at releasing these hormones. In others words, you need regular exercise to get the full effect.

Here's a few tips. If you join a gym then go in the morning and choose a gym within eight minutes of home. The chances of you still going after the first month are seven times better if you follow those two guidelines. Secondly, if you get too carried away and end up as a sweaty strained puddle on the floor then your brain will try and put you off going in future. After all, your deep seated instincts are usually trying to protect you from pain. If you think about the gym and your heart sinks then you won't go. As I said previously; try bite sized, attainable, tasks; the same is definitely true of exercise. Make life into a series of short sprints not a marathon.

Better still though, try and get exercise that is more fun. Try and drum up someone to play tennis with or Sunday morning football or borrow a dog to walk or coming to think of it you could even advertise yourself as a paid dog walker.

A colleague of mine once placed an ad in the local newspaper. It said 'I'm 25 and new in the area. Is there anyone out there who wants to practice beginner's tennis or ten pin bowling?' She felt very self conscious doing it, but made two good friends in this manner, and subsequently mentioned to a friend of hers what she'd done and they replied, 'Why didn't you tell me? I would love to drive over on a Saturday morning and do something like that with you. It would be a chance to meet up.' Win win win.

Assuming you haven't just jumped up and gone off for a run or dashed up to the gym, let's get a bit of exercise now.

Stand up.

Look at the time, and then dance around the room in a reasonably energetic manner for three whole minutes.

Or skip or jog on the spot.

Did you do that? No? Please don't waste everyone's time making me use another page to drone on about motivation.

A word about self hypnosis. There are a number of good books out there that can teach you simple techniques that are likely to benefit you, and some of the self help books even have a hypnotic CD in the back cover. I can't cover it in detail, not least because it would unbalance the book. But as a taster for this sort of thing why not try the following exercise.

Firstly pick an objective or goal, possibly something that can be measured, like how long you go in the morning without a cigarette, or feeling more positive about yourself, or feeling less anxious in certain situations.

You must not fall asleep – after all you are effectively talking to yourself, so no nodding off please. You are trying to get very relaxed and suggestible. Here's a simple example of what to say to yourself once comfortable...

'I am in a lift. The lift is on the ground floor. Soon the lift will drop gently down below ground to level one. When it drops gently down to level one I will feel more and more relaxed. It is now dropping down to level one, as it drops down I am feeling more and more relaxed. I am going deeper and deeper. I am now feeling more and more relaxed.'

Repeat the same internal speech for level two, then level three, then level four.

You might now say to yourself, 'I am so deeply relaxed... that my mind has become sensitive... so receptive to everything I say... every day I will become more alert...

more wide awake... I will become much less easily tired... much less fatigued... much less discouraged. Every day I will become so deeply interested in what I am doing... so deeply interested in whatever is going on... that my mind is much less preoccupied with myself... every day my mind will become calmer and clearer...'

You might now want to add the objective that you thought about earlier on this page.

Yes, there's more to hypnosis than this but start practising this until your book arrives.

POST NATAL DEPRESSION, REDUNDANCY, BREAK-UPS, BEING IN PRISON, BEREAVEMENT AND MORE...

Why on earth have I lumped these very different problems together? After all, Post Natal Depression definitely has a metabolic or hormonal element and is so complicated it would need its own book, so what hare-brained tangent am I off on now? Let me explain... starting with prison camps.

Imagine a generic prison camp from history: it doesn't matter what country or era you choose. What is the standard practice when they treat prisoners? They would probably take away their normal clothes and make them all dress the same. They might give them numbers instead of names. They certainly take away their day jobs and make them do menial work such as cleaning or working in a chain gang. They restrict face to face access to their friends and family. They reduce their communication with the outside world, and in the case of solitary confinement they reduce communication to zero. All these measures have something in common: they take away our identity.

We gain our identities and express our identities through our jobs, our clothes, who we spend time with and how we communicate with people. When these elements are taken away it is a punishment or even a torture.

Now consider having a baby. You have spent your teenage years and early adulthood slowly discovering who you are: forging your identity and expressing it in what you do, how you look and how you behave. Until you had a child you might have defined yourself by your work, or by your friendships or your nights out with the girls or whatever; you might have seen yourself as a 'career woman' or 'part of a successful team' or 'the life and soul of the party' or 'a head turner' or 'someone who was always there for her friends' – suddenly you're stuck on a dull Tuesday morning with nothing but some kid's TV to watch and a buggy to push through the rain. You have literally lost your identity.

You no longer have daily access to your colleagues, you are no longer treated the same way by people, and because children can be messy and your figure changes when you are pregnant, you may even have to wear different clothes. You are forced to do menial jobs and answer to the demands of an irrational dictator (your toddler): in short the situation has an alarming amount in common with prison and a lot of the 'torture' of this is to do with your loss of identity.

A similar train of thought can be applied to the loss of a friendship or spouse through divorce or bereavement. As the relationship passes, so you lose a little of 'who you were.'

So, what can we do? A variation of one of the earlier exercises, basically.

Find your list of personal strengths that you made earlier.

Get another piece of paper and draw up five favourite ways to pass your time.

Spend a while thinking how you can 'express' the person you truly are a little better.

And here's a thought you perhaps should add to the equation...

Imagine your character and lifestyle are like a well-loved CD by a singer or band that you like. There are a dozen or more tracks on the CD and you probably have some favourite tracks that you play more often than the rest: perhaps they were the hit singles. Think of your favourite pastimes as being those favourite tracks. While you are pregnant you may not get a chance to play those favourite tracks very often, but instead you may get the chance to explore other tracks, other aspects of you, that have been there all along, but which up until now have seemed less important. Childcare takes up about ten years out of the seventy years we may spend on the planet. There are sixty years to play the tracks you like. In the meantime relish the chance to explore those less obvious parts of yourself. Perhaps you used to organise the office; now you may have to organise the PTA. Perhaps you used to be a teacher; now you may have a chance to do the reading you've always meant to do. The key thing to remember is that when you are playing the other tracks on the CD the favourite tracks don't magically cease to exist: they will be there all along for you to return to one day.

And as for losing relationships...

We're all only human, of course. But some human traits are less useful than others. One is the way we can dwell on the negative.

Two friends are talking.

'I saw a fantastic film the other day,' says one. 'It was gripping and fun and romantic and exhilarating. It was awful.'

'What on earth do you mean?' asks the other friend.

'It was an absolutely perfect film but, you see, it ended.'

'Ah,' sympathises the friend. 'I know what you mean. I read a book the other week. It was so *me*. It was probably the best book I will ever read. I put so much emotional investment into it, and so much of my time and effort, but I wish I had never started reading it now, because it ended. Of course I realise now that no matter what I did, it was going to end. I feel such a fool for ever believing otherwise.'

The two friends look sympathetically at each other and sigh.

What's wrong with that conversation? Everything, obviously, yet when we say, 'I loved that *relationship* and I put everything into it, but it ended. It's really messed me up,' we think that is a reasonable thing to say. So that's the first tip. If you have been dwelling on a break-up, close your eyes and think of three stand out moments from that relationship; three great things you did together. Really imagine them carefully, one by one. Visualise the scene and enjoy its details. If you had had your time again, no matter how it all ended, would you really pass up on those moments? If, conversely, you are struggling to think of three good times with that person then give yourself a talking to: he or she is not worth a moment more of your time.

Now get a clean sheet of paper and stare at it. Picture that person's face on the piece of paper. If they have done you wrong, then they are looking at you and they are saying 'Sorry'. See their lips say the word. Now they are closing their eyes and their face is shrinking. It is getting smaller and smaller and fading in colour.

Now fold up the piece of paper and crumple it up tight and throw it in the bin.

Now think of another person from your life who you like or liked. It could be a recent friend or someone you knew when you were five. Now think of an incident where you really enjoyed yourself with them. Picture it brightly. Laughing with them, talking with them.

Now picture someone else you like; someone in your present who is only half important to you, perhaps someone with whom you have a different kind of friendship: a relative perhaps or a colleague or acquaintance who you get on with okay, but you are not very close to. Appreciate this relationship for exactly what it is. Cordial but not intense. Helpful but not overbearing. A laugh, but not deep. Thoughtful, rather than frivolous. Now repeat the process with another person who is not that close to you. It is not that these people will necessarily ever be that important for you, it is more that we are well served when we diversify our attitudes towards relationships.

There's an old saying about relationships: a man looks at his wife and wishes she was still the girl he married. A woman marries a man and sets about trying to change him. Both attitudes are wrong.

Sometimes we should enjoy every relationship for exactly what it is at the time. No more and no less.

Another huge element of losing a relationship is that people suddenly get it into their heads that they may never date again and that they don't know where their future lies, and looking to the future is also a key element of this book. Where does your future lie? I have no idea. But, one of the many themes of this book is that you have more chance of getting an interesting future if you diversify your interests and get out more.

So... you will need another piece of paper. Again, I make no apologies for this; by the end of this book I want you to end up with several pieces of paper, all full of positive information and all pointing the way forward.

On this new piece of paper I want you to list five things you would like to do but which you haven't got round to recently or indeed ever. It might be things like 'Take up painting' or 'Learn some Spanish' or 'Ring up that old friend I haven't seen since college,' or 'Learn salsa dancing,' or 'Support the local team more often.' There may be evening classes you can do or a local group of enthusiasts you can join; it may involve a few phone calls or a hunt around the net. The net result is that you should be cultivating a few extra hobbies than you strictly have time for. Why? Because no matter how clever you are, over the course of seventy years there will be patches of your life which will run into trouble. Your career can't possibly be perfect month in month out, and neither can your relationships, so you need a few extra interests which you can switch your mind to from time to time.

Once you've decided on your list of five interests, leave it out in plain view.

A final word about losing a relationship. The ones that hurt the most are often the ones where we fell deeply in love, obviously, so it can be very useful to recognise in ourselves the reasons why we personally fall in love and a lot of people *subconsciously* fall in love when they are *subconsciously* wondering where their future lies. The summer before leaving home as a teenager, or the first year at university are common times to fall in love. Or in a Professor Higgins style we can sometimes fall in love with someone who has a lot to teach us. Or in a Pretty Woman style, we can fall in love with someone glamorous or successful or famous or moneyed, because they can offer us an intro into another way of life. Does this sound cynical? Yes, of course it does, but would Pretty Woman have been the same film if Richard Gere had been a rubbish collector? My point is that is we have brains that sometimes steer us towards our futures by using sneaky tricks like making us fall in love. If we have a brain that tends to do this it is more likely to be a bigger blow when that relationship falls apart because the very element we were craving – a future – has been taken away from us. We are a lot happier if we can recognise these traits in ourselves and see them in perspective.

This concept also helps us to understand why we sometimes have an 'out of the frying pan and into the fire' mentality. Perhaps our job is in the doldrums, so we fall in love with the idea of having children or moving abroad. Mysteriously we don't worry about the endless practical problems and drop in living standard this will entail, but we do see the practical problems in our current life as insurmountable and irritating. Why? Because we've seen our future and fallen in love with it. This is not to say that we should never have children or move abroad or fall in love, it is just a whole lot healthier if we see these desires for exactly what they are, and enjoy them for exactly what they are. As I am very fond of pointing out, no ONE solution will change your life 100% and that includes moving abroad, marrying or having children: understand that and you are less likely to jump from a frying pan to a fire.

Just as importantly:

NO ONE **PERSON** WILL CHANGE OUR LIVES 100%

Saying, 'Oh if only I had a boyfriend/girlfriend' or 'I wish I still had X or Y in my life' is largely a waste of time. Even if that person was indeed perfect, it is not their job to make your life better.

Read this out loud; it is one of the most important sentences in the entire book:

IT IS NOT SOMEONE ELSE'S JOB TO MAKE ME HAPPY.

Cover it up with your hand and see if you can still say it out loud. Like every piece of advice in this book, this will be more relevant to some people than to others, but I would bet that at some stage in all of our lives we have, deep down, blamed our lives on other people. A good rule of thumb is to wonder for a second, 'Is there anyone I have been repeatedly obsessing about?' It is not their job to make you happy. It is not your partner's job, it is not your boss's job, it is not your colleague's job, it is not your friend's job, it is not your parents' job. Even Doctors, Psychiatrists and myself... we can offer tips and advice, we can highlight research and share our experience, but it's not our job to make you happy.

It's up to you to be happy

A quick word about status...

Apparently people who win Oscars go on to live an average of five years longer than their fellow actors who were only Oscar nominees. Amazing, isn't it? This might of course simply be a statistical quirk, but equally it may go to show what a boost to our health some external validation and extra status can bring us.

Status is a peculiar, but very important concept. Have you ever been on holiday in Greece or wherever and met a barman or barwoman who lives out there temporarily. They are sunny and relaxed and enjoying their summer. They probably earn a fraction of what you do and live in a tiny flat and rarely buy new clothes. And yet you envied them. Or perhaps something similar has happened as you considered a gardener pottering around the local park or a librarian with an apparently simple job. The moral? A lot of us would be very happy with simpler lives but we are just so hung up on our relative status, possessions, career and success. Perhaps we need to rethink the balance a bit.

When was the last time you felt envious of someone in your life? Think about that person and their whole lifestyle. Would you actually want all of their life, or have you just focussed on one element of it, that reflects on your needs? Is there any way you could perhaps adopt a little of that one element and incorporate it into your lifestyle?

Now focus on three people one by one who are less fortunate than yourself. If you are struggling to do this, it might be more effective to think about the people you have left behind over the years. For example, you may be struggling at college, but what about the people from your class who didn't even make it as far as you? What did they go on to do?

Now think of three countries around the world where people are in a worse position than you. How do they live? What do they eat? What do they earn?

Now think of three situations in recent history where people in your own country had difficult lives.

Now clear your mind and change tack completely. Quickly list in your head all the things you have done in the last week. Little jobs, like tidying or cheering up a friend or finishing a piece of work; now add big achievements from the past like buying a car or a house or holidays you have gone on, or a job you managed to get by beating other candidates. Now think of all the exams you have ever passed, including your driving test and each and every GCSE. Now think of all the things you have done for other people: made meals for the kids, organised a birthday treat for a friend? Now think of things that you have enjoyed: films seen, nights out. This is who you are. It's not bad is it?

Tonight as you are falling asleep you need to repeat this phrase to yourself three times. Then a few minutes later say it to yourself three times again. Then a few minutes after that, do it again.

Whenever I see the colour red I am going to be overwhelmed with happiness.

In the meantime, close your eyes and place your hands on your lap with your fingers interlocked. Say this phrase in your head three lots of three times.

Another thing to do before you go to sleep is to think of three things that happened that day which were good. These should relate to your senses.

• Something that *tasted* good.

• Something that *looked* good or pleasing or fun.

• Something that you *heard* that was good, or pleasing or fun.

Again you should practice this now, choosing something from today, or possibly the last couple of days.

Imagine your old age; imagine being seventy or older.

Imagine looking back at the age you are now. What would you advise yourself now that you can see this year in the context of a whole lifetime? What would you think of the decisions you are making? Give yourself some advice.

Let's take a moment to catch our breath and recap the general message of all of this.

The brain is an organ like any other bodily organ, and like any organ it can get damaged. In many ways it is also like a muscle, in that it is a 'doing' organ that can be used for many different functions. To help a bodily organ or damaged muscle we can:

1 Remove factors that are harming it.

2 Give it exercise.

3 Give it the right environmental factors.

4 Give it the right nutrition.

Nutrition is covered next, but to recap the first three. To help with removing the factors that have harmed the brain we have been looking at how we can see relationships and problems in a new light and looking at how we spend our time to see how we can have more of what we enjoy and less of what is annoying us.

To the give the brain exercise I have taken us through a number of mental exercises, ranging from visualisation exercises to hypnosis and cognitive therapy style exercises.

On the subject of creating the right environment I have been suggesting everything from good music to diversifying your pastimes to strengthening your relationships.

No ONE cure will change your life 100%, but you can easily make fifty changes that will each change your life 2%.

You might think I have stressed that last one enough times; after all, it is patently the basis of the entire book. Unbelievably however, people say to me every single day of my life, 'Yeah, I like your train of thought, but tell me, what's the answer?' or 'I've read your stuff, but I get so depressed, what should I do?' Aaaaaaah! There IS no one answer. Just follow the instructions and actually carry out the tasks. Yes there will be bad days as well as good days, but the trend will be up.

... AND DRINK

Nutrition: I personally don't think you can eat the right things and expect it to cure depression.

However, I *do* believe that if you eat and drink badly it can cause depression or make it worse. Eat and drink badly and you are fighting the battle with one hand tied behind your back.

Let's start with the obvious one: alcohol.

Alcohol is a depressant. It depresses brain function.

I will say that again: alcohol is a depressant. It depresses brain function.

People tend to think alcohol is a stimulant because it depresses their inhibitions and they associate it with parties, fun times and Friday nights, but make no mistake; alcohol works by *blocking* receptors in the brain not stimulating them. It causes the level of brain activity to be depressed. What's more, normally for every thought we have our brain comes up with a few alternative thoughts to balance it and help check its validity. Alcohol tends to block these alternative thoughts so that we have a less balanced view of life. That is why after a few drinks, sad ideas will easily make us maudlin.

What is the alcoholic's mantra? 'Poor me. Poor me. Pour me a drink.' A huge number of alcoholics are essentially masking their depression with another, bigger problem: booze. Booze itself makes them more depressed.

And then there is the hangover. A really bad week of depression can be set off by one morning's hangover alone. And don't get me started on the subject of drugs... dope doesn't just block brain receptors; it *kills off* entire neural pathways.

We all know alcohol is a pest and we all know the sorts of measures that help. If you are a depressive you are going to need to take alcohol seriously. Obviously there are social pressures involved, but if you're going out for the evening, how about making sure your first drink is non-alcoholic, or make sure that every other drink is non-alcoholic, or simply choose drinks with lower alcohol content. Or here is a great tip that even saves money... when it is your friend's round then have bottle of lager, but when it is your turn to buy a round, then choose a coke or tonic for yourself. People won't notice and they get the fun of being generous.

Here's a quick test:

You are ordering a drink and the bartender replies, 'Would you like the house double, it's only fifty pence more?'

What do you reply?

Correct. The answer is 'No thank you, I'm fine.'

It's worth remembering that 'House Double' is in fact code for 'Some cheap knock-off spirit the landlord's mate brought from abroad in the back of his van.'

One lengthy study about alcohol had a very interesting finding. The top two factors that give people a hangover are a) how much you drink (what a surprise) and b) how tiring your week has been.

This isn't so amazing, but what I found interesting was that how chronically tired you are is *equally* important in creating a bad hangover. Often at the end of a long week, that is precisely when we haven't got the energy to look after ourselves and cook, and it is all too easy to have several drinks to 'unwind'.

Another study about alcohol showed that a lot of early evening drinking is actually caused by *hunger*. You have a long day at work and by 6pm you haven't eaten for five hours. Your body notices the low sugar levels in your blood stream and motivates you to provide it with carbohydrates. A wine, a lager, a vodka and tonic... they all have sugars in them.

The study showed clearly that if you keep some nuts at work and eat a handful before leaving the office then you are half as likely to have a drink in the next two hours.

Chocolate

Thinking more on what we all eat... sugar rushes are bad news. Too much chocolate and snacking and coke, and your sugar levels are flying all over the place. It's like the country's economy; if house prices or inflation or employment are flying all over the place then it's stressful and debilitating. Or it's like driving a car but cutting off the petrol then injecting too much. You can insert your own analogy, basically. It's the same for your brain: if you are overloading it with fuel and then suddenly cutting off the supply again what good is that going to do? Proper food, regularly eaten. It's not that hard. You don't see athletes eating sweets; they eat real food, like pasta and rice. Complex carbohydrates, not simple sugars. It's not hard to eat an apple or banana and drink a glass of semi-skimmed milk.

Chocolate in particular contains drugs that affect your mood and make your brain addicted. One famous finding is that when people are treated for drug addiction by using drugs that stop their craving for opiates, they also go off eating chocolate. Go figure.

Vegetarianism

The average vegetarian lives longer than the average omnivore. I say this to point out that I am not against vegetarianism, but I am just about to make myself unpopular by pointing out something very important about completely avoiding meat.

One of the most important chemicals in the brain that makes us happy is Serotonin. To make Serotonin, your brain needs a protein that simply does not exist in the vegetable world. It is no coincidence therefore that one study showed that vegetarians have lower levels of Serotonin in their brains. Another study showed that vegetarians are ten per cent more likely to suffer from chronic depression. This is not very surprising, when you consider that human brains evolved for hundreds of thousands of years with a diet that included proteins from the animal world. It is probably very wise therefore to eat more eggs and a wider variety of nuts than at first seems likely.

So those were some possible don'ts; alcohol, chocolate and sweets. Here are some more positive ways at looking at nutrition...

A good project for today and tomorrow is to learn some new recipes. We all do it: we spot an interesting recipe in a magazine or we leaf through the new Jamie Oliver book but we never quite get round to new recipes unless we have guests.

A resolution worth trying is to learn a new simple recipe a week. If you live with someone they will be impressed, not least because it looks like tangible evidence that you are putting some effort in to cheer yourself up and get your act together. It certainly conforms to our previous objective of finding bite-sized tasks to do which have a quantifiable outcome. Bite-sized... it was very nearly a decent pun.

Something I do when I go round the supermarket (yes I'm a bloke and yes I do the household shopping every week: the only difference is that when a man does it, he expects praise) is to go to the section where they sell recipe books and I prop one open at an interesting recipe then go round the supermarket to buy the ingredients. I then replace the book on the shelf having made a note of any technique in the recipe I might easily forget. It's cheap, simple and effective.

However, not only am I suggesting we all learn some recipes, but there are some ingredients worth using that *may* improve depression.

There is some research that shows that a chemical called chromium picolinate, a trace mineral naturally found in mushrooms, liver, whole grains and many other foods, has significant effects on people suffering from the most common sorts of depression. The relevant depressions were characterized by a need for extra sleep, carbohydrate cravings, and being over sensitive to rejection. Such depressions respond to a class of antidepressants known as monoamine oxidase inhibitors, but these drugs carry with them dietary restrictions as well as side effects like sexual dysfunction and weight gain. Why not try and drum up some recipes that involve mushrooms, or pate or whole grains? It can't be that hard.

Here are some other views on nutrition born out by research...

Meals that are balanced and contain complex carbohydrates, protein and fat will slowly fuel our brain chemicals throughout the day. It is the ideal way to keep our brains in balance during any stressful patches that may be around the corner.

Complex carbohydrates, such as pastas, noodles, rice and potatoes increase the amount of serotonin in your brain. As well as being a 'happy chemical' it is thought that it boosts your mood, calms you down and helps you sleep. Fruits, vegetables and whole grains are all good at providing complex carbohydrates, so it doesn't just have to be the starchy foods.

Protein-rich foods help to slow down the rate at which sugar is released into your bloodstream and keeps your blood sugar balanced. It also keeps you feeling full longer, making you less likely to grab for a high-calorie sweet snack. Nutritional sources for this include dairy foods, fish, meats, legumes (beans and lentils), peanut butter, poultry and tofu.

So-called 'Essential Fats' (e.g. omega-6 and omega-3 fatty acids) help the flow of nutrients into cells and furthermore they allow waste products to escape from the cells. Salmon and other oily fish such as sardines and tuna contain omega-3 fatty acids, which appear to help relieve mild depression. Other food sources include nuts such as almonds and walnuts, oils such as canola, flax, and soybean, and seeds such as flax and pumpkin.

The following is the tip that over the years has caused the most disagreement, so have a read and consider the concept, you can be for or against it but either way it is so important you should certainly have *thought* about it...

I went through a phase of being fascinated by a certain kind of book and I read about six of them in a row. The books in question were written by women who had recovered from eating disorders or depression or drug abuse or alcoholism and were telling us all about their life. I was interested to see if these people had any traits in common, (apart from a desire to harm themselves, obviously).

One thing that struck me between the eyes was that these people all hated their own company. If you put them in a room on their own, they would just get more ill. This ties in with my earlier point about solitary confinement; most people see being stuck on their own as a punishment.

It wasn't just that these people needed other people; they also tended to obsessively compare themselves to other people. Were other women in the room better looking than them? Were they doing better than them? Were they getting more attention? Were they better dressed? Did they have more friends?

I fundamentally believe that if you enjoy your own company then you yourself are happy and free from depression. To broaden it out a bit: if you like your own company; if you like yourself; if you don't compare yourself to others; if you are happy for others when they do well…. then you yourself will feel the happiest person alive.

I am not saying you should renounce friendship. I am saying you should enjoy friendship and being on your own as two separate and distinct joys.

I don't think any of this is the least bit controversial, but you would be amazed how many people have been really fierce in telling me I am 'wrong.' One person, quite reasonably, wrote to me to say he took a long hiking trip on his own and half way through a six hour coach trip he literally went insane. There are other tales of people who have gone into an 'isolation tank' and the lack of external stimulus gave them a psychotic episode. I totally agree. My point is not 'isolate yourself and you will be happy' but if and when you can learn to love being on your own, then you will be happy.

Have you ever gone to a restaurant and eaten on your own? Have you every gone to a cinema on your own? Statistically you probably haven't. People do sit in their sitting room and watch a TV on their own but they would rather miss a film they are desperate to see than be *seen* to go alone to a cinema. Presumably it's social conditioning of some sort. People don't actually stare and point at you if you eat a meal on your own or see the latest movie; it just feels like they do. It is all in our heads.

'BUY' A DAY OF HAPPINESS

Whether or not you agree with this concept...

Book a trip, book a theatre, gig, or an outing. If you're on a tight budget, hunt out something free: galleries, groups playing in bars, open mike comedy nights. Preferably something different to what you usually choose to do. I live near London, so it's only an example: sometimes I hop on the train and select six galleries and gigs to see (in this week's Time Out 507 free ideas are listed. 507!) I take all six 'on the run' why? Because often something doesn't live up to expectations and you don't want to pin your day out on one of those because that would be a downer and besides, rushing around is a bit of exercise. It is far better than sitting at home, and for the reasons given on the previous page I would suggest you should think about doing the outing on your own.

Here is a conversation I bet you have never heard:

'This is absolutely astonishing. The most amazing thing. A bunch of complete strangers have decided to spend tens of thousands of pounds on me. They have paid for a team of people to come and talk to me one by one, week after week for years; they tell me about stuff they have learnt in Universities, they demonstrate stuff and show me skills; all so that I can then go off to have a better life and become rich!'

'Ah,' you reply. 'Yes, I've heard of that. It's called state funded education. Most people moan about it.'

In contrast, here are some conversations we hear all too often:

'Every night I have a battle with my teenagers to get them to do their homework.'

'Oh that lesson is so boring,' says a school kid. 'That teacher keeps setting us more and more work to do and expecting us to read around the subject. It is so not going to happen.'

And it's not just education where we have a crazy attitude.

'I want to be fit and healthy, and live a long productive life. But I keep putting cigarettes in my mouth.'

'I want to be slim, but I keep buying chocolate and French Fries.'

'I want to be happy, but I keep moping around the house dwelling on my problems.'

We keep seeing life as a battle with us on the losing, aggrieved side. It starts in childhood with us versus a parent, then it might become us versus a school teacher, then us versus an irritating boss or colleague or spouse or 'difficult' child. In fact we get so hooked on having battles that as adults we end up having battles with ourselves about eating, exercise, smoking, spending money and, you name it basically.

In fact, let's face it, I have been so sure that this is a universal trait that I have assumed that you, as a reader, would be happy with the whole premise that we could see depression as an enemy that we can fight and overcome. This is a fine concept when it is *useful*, but when seeing life as a battle is destructive and time consuming it may be better to not see situations as conflicts. In other words, only see a situation as a battle when it is in your *interests* to do so.

Some people reading this book will even see this as a chance to have an imaginary battle with *me*. Their heads will be full of thoughts like, 'Ah he's wrong because...' or 'Well I went jogging a few times, but nothing happened.' Or 'I've tried things like this before, well I didn't actually do the exercises but...' or 'Oh he seems to be claiming it's all in the mind and if I just had a different attitude then...'

It's as if some people need to prove to themselves and others that they are incurable, and the way of doing this is to take issue with anyone who suggests remedies.

Certainly if you don't try a remedy it *certainly* won't work, so it's convenient for these people not to try in the first place.

As for the complaint that I am claiming depression is 'all the mind' or that people are somehow 'choosing' to be depressed (another common moan from readers) I actually have a lot of sympathy. In a very literal sense, of course, depression *is* all in the mind. The mind is the organ that has the illness; what people don't want to be told is that they just have to magically snap out of it. That is no more logical than telling a torn strained muscle to snap out of it.

On the other hand, think of your brain as a machine in a box. Most of us have become depressed purely by the input that has gone into our brain. It is not as if we have *physically* put anything in our brain. The only things that ever went into our brain were thoughts. So we can all agree that thoughts can make us depressed. Why do we struggle with the concept that having the right thoughts can slowly but surely make us happy? Because...

Depression is an illness that robs people of their belief that people can cure it.

I totally agree that we do not choose to be depressed, but we *do* choose what we think about all day. After all, I'm sure we can all agree that if we dwell on gloomy thoughts all day we will become gloomy. Why can't we accept the opposite may also be true? If we think happy thoughts all day, we *will* become happy.

In fact (cynics get ready to heckle now):

If you think happy thoughts all day, then you ARE happy.

There's an old light bulb joke that is still funny after all these years.

'How many psychiatrists does it take to change a light bulb?'

'Only one. But the light bulb has really got to want to change.'

If you really want to be happy then throw yourself into all the reasonable options available. Taking fifty actions to improve your mood by 2% is not difficult and it is not far fetched to believe that it will improve your life. In fact, it strains credulity to believe that it won't make a difference. If you let your depression persuade you it is a better use of your time sitting around feeling sorry for yourself and endlessly telling yourself you are a hopeless case then good luck with that. It is far less likely to work than the fifty suggestions in this book. Why would anyone kid themselves otherwise?

So:

This book is not a battle. It is not a trial of strength. This book is just a learning tool. It is just a useful pile of tips that will beat your depression and change your life forever. There is no battle. Your relationship with a teacher is not a trial of strength, your relationship with your child or partner or boss or me is not a trial of strength.

And that leads us to the task in this chapter. Have a little think about your life – at home, at work, at school – and check whether or not you are engaged in 'fake battles.' Do you find yourself having a trial of strength with your partner over who did the chores or who did the most childcare or who spent the most money? Do you find you get into a power struggle with your boss or colleagues or your mother? Or rows with your children about tidying their rooms or doing their homework or eating their food?

Battles are debilitating and even in the rare cases where they are genuine, they are rarely worth taking on unless you are going to win them. As for the others... just let go. I know too many people whose lives are ruled by their alleged battles with their teenagers or spouse or boss. Let it go! Let it wash over you.

The next two sections may help in different ways...

Here is a list of how we sometimes deal with difficulties in relationships and issues at work.

- I get resentful.
- I dwell on grievances.
- I sulk.
- I am not the first to forgive and forget.
- I tend to take things personally.
- There are colleagues who irritate me.
- I co-operate less with the person afterward conflict.
- I moan.
- I get petty.
- I get angry.

Here is another list of ways in which we sometimes deal with the same problems.

- I just let it wash over me.
- I can see that a lot of people would find it irritating but I prefer to chill.
- I see the funny side of it.
- I take it on the chin and move on.
- I am big and warm and capable about it all.
- I didn't even notice there was a problem, I was busy doing something useful.
- If other people want to be petty; let them get on with it.
- I sleep on it and in the morning I can see a number of solutions that make sense.

- I take a bit of time out and get on with something else useful instead.

- I like to feel I help a little and give and not expect any praise or anything in return.

- I can see that the other person might be under a lot of stress at the moment.

Now think of someone you admire. Someone you would like to be, perhaps. George Clooney? J K Rowling? Margaret Thatcher? Richard Branson? Catherine Zeta Jones? Bill Gates? It really doesn't matter, so long as it is someone you truly admire.

Now look at the two lists of traits above. Which list do you associate with them? Which list would you like to associate with yourself? It is tempting to think that someone like Richard Branson can 'afford' to be good natured because he has money, but what about when he started his business using only a public payphone and some catalogues printed at the local copy centre? What about when George Clooney was in the film Attack of the Killer Tomatoes or had one or two lines a week in the sitcom Roseanne? Which list of traits would have helped them progress up through life? The positive list. If they had indulged in being a seething bag of resentment who blamed others for their life and dwelled on their problems, would they have gone on to do so well?

The task in this section is simple. Choose which of those two lists you would like to be.

Breathing is a reflection of the level of tension in your body. When you are all stressed up, your breathing may become rapid and shallow, and occurs high up in the chest. When you feel relaxed the opposite occurs: you breathe fully and deeply, and from lower down: your abdomen.

Take just three minutes to do this breathing exercise and you will instantly feel relaxed.

Place one palm on your abdomen right beneath your rib cage. Now breathe in deeply through your nose into the very bottom of your lungs. Really send that air deep down: as *low* as you can. You should be able to feel your hand actually rise as you breathe in. Your rib cage should move only the smallest amount while your abdomen expands.

Now that you have taken in a full breath, pause for a moment and then exhale slowly through your nose. Really let that breath out deeply and completely. As you let the breath out, allow your whole body to just let go. Feel your arms relax and slump down. Feel your shoulders relax and slump down. Then after that, make them slump down even more.

Now stay slumped and 'breathed out' and count to five in a relaxed manner.

Now start all over again.

Do the whole thing ten times over. A bit like the hypnosis exercise where you went down in an imaginary lift:

imagine each breathing cycle is another stage taking you lower and lower, and more relaxed.

Make sure to practice this over the days ahead so that you can use it at a moment's notice; when you need to unwind, just let go, and let life wash over you.

Now try another very simple breathing exercise...

When we breathe out, our pulse is slower than when we breathe in. So sit up straight and keep your shoulders back but relaxed. Rest your hands on your lap with your fingers interlocked. Now slowly but evenly let the air out of your lungs while gently holding in your stomach. Do this for a good minute with your breathing out taking twice as long as your breathing in. Slower breathing also means your lungs have more time to remove carbon dioxide and carbon monoxide from your bloodstream.

As with other exercises where I have asked you to interlock your fingers, you will start to associate doing this with feeling relaxed. If in the months to come you need to relax, then place your hands on your lap with your fingers interlocked and you will feel more relaxed instantly. You can combine this with any of the breathing or other relaxation exercises. Your mood will improve instantly.

If you get a day where you feel low, try and work out roughly what time you started dwelling on your problems or at what time your mood lowered. How long did that patch then last? Twenty minutes? Four hours? Try and put a rough time to it, and then plan how you can now spend the exact same length of time doing something enjoyable. The time could be spend day dreaming or making lists of your all time favourite films, or chatting to someone you have been meaning to catch up with, or reading a book or going out to the cinema or hooking up with someone or having a hot bath. It doesn't matter what the task is, so long as you make sure you have given yourself time 'off' from thinking about whatever it was that bugged you earlier.

It's nice to be nice and you can't have too many friends. Think about a person in your life. Consider what they often talk about. Consider what interests them. Now think of something interesting to say on a subject that interests them, perhaps a question. When in conversation, people like to have a chance to breathe. It sounds silly and little but when they speak let them get to the end of their sentences, and then count to two or three before speaking yourself. Keep consistent eye contact. Smile and show interest in what they are saying. Don't sit with your arms crossed over your chest: if in doubt, take your cue from the other person's body language or sit with 'open' body language without invading the other person's space.

39 WHAT AM I ON ABOUT NOW?

There are a couple of interesting studies that fly against our gut instincts about conversations. One study showed that if you get someone to talk about themselves, then they find *us* interesting. The second study was carried out at parties. They measured laughter, the amount that people talked over each other, and they measured how loudly people talked. The same people were then asked afterwards how much they enjoyed the party. Amazingly, most people reported they had enjoyed the parties that had *less* laughter, less overlapping conversation and the less voluble chat. So the recipe for people enjoying themselves seems to be; relax and let people express themselves.

We all like to be liked, and we all like other people to enjoy themselves, and we all like other people to enjoy our company. Sometimes these very simple solutions mentioned above are all it takes.

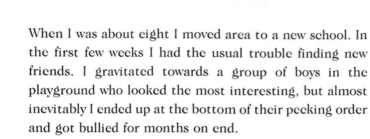

When I was about eight I moved area to a new school. In the first few weeks I had the usual trouble finding new friends. I gravitated towards a group of boys in the playground who looked the most interesting, but almost inevitably I ended up at the bottom of their pecking order and got bullied for months on end.

I finally mentioned this to an adult and a day or so later a teacher made a simple suggestion. She pointed out a lad I hadn't noticed before and suggested we played together. We got on really well and formed a great friendship. No doubt he was also someone who didn't fit in. From that very instant onwards I was happy. I was even treated well by the bullies from then on, and went on to become best friends with one of them, without any further trouble. What are the morals here? There are many. There were several hundred kids in that school but inexplicably I was drawn the very ones who made my life a misery. The key to my happiness was in my hands all along. A small but important change was all it took. By not being so interested in the 'smart set' they were, paradoxically, more interested in me.

The reason I mention it, is that bullying is a very common cause of depression, as are anxieties in general. Stresses at work, financial problems, someone who is making themselves feel better by putting us down: these are all major causes of depression.

Have a little review of your life. Is there one big factor that is the cause of a lot of anxiety? You may want to look at the 'to do' list you made earlier and see what *sort* of problems you are finding mostly stressful. Do you perhaps need to talk to someone about these problems, just as I did when I was eight? Perhaps you need to remove yourself from these situations more, or even explain to a person the effect they are having on you? Like my story of bullying there might be one key change that will remove a huge amount of anxiety from your life. Obviously, if this happens to be a big change like, say, changing jobs you need to weigh it up carefully and consider the 'out of the frying pan into the fire' type concerns I mentioned earlier and as I keep saying, any change should be part of a larger package because (all together now) we mustn't keep assuming that just one change will improve our lives 100%.

Now for a little more background on the thinking behind the strategy we are pursuing on these pages.

The vast majority of the emails I got via my websites were from two main groups of people.

The first big group were younger people – 17 to about 24 year olds. Frequently their underlying problem seemed to be a general anxiety about the future. On some level they were daunted by the enormity of it all. How were they ever going to get ahead enough to have a decent job, house, relationships, a glamorous lifestyle or whatever else they had in mind? In other words they couldn't see where their future lay or a realistic way of getting there.

The second most common group of people who wrote to me were older: 30 to 50 year olds. They were often depressed because they were effectively asking 'Is this it?' They were looking at their time consuming children or their tight budget or their same-old job or their so-so relationships and they felt that for them the music had stopped and this was the total of their future.

In many ways this is the same problem but for a different age group, and it all relates to our expectations of life. With the twenty-somethings who write to me, I am often surprised by their level of barely-suppressed panic and I always want to say, 'You're only young; you've got a lifetime to slowly realise your various dreams.' But there's not much point saying that because for some reason no one truly believes they are young. I, myself, can remember panicking about turning 25: if a forty year old had told me I was only young and to stop worrying, my reaction would be that they 'simply didn't understand.'

I don't know about everyone else, but I found being in my twenties was very over-rated. You are stuck in the lower foothills of your career, your bills seem disproportionately high and everything seems such a slog. And yet we live in a culture that pedals the notion that being in your twenties is the ideal age: we were told it would be a time of glamorous dates, travel, freedom and success.

Sex and the City is a good example of how we acquire our ideas: we imagine we should be eating at the best restaurants, having cocktails in the trendiest bars and wearing the latest clothes. We should have thrilling jobs and be invited to the openings of major New York clubs and galleries, and all the while we should have a circle of devoted friends who will, in the words of the theme tune to Friends 'Be there for you.' We know deep down that in real life the characters in Sex and the City would all have been sacked for endlessly having brunch during what should be their work hours, but somehow we still cling on to the idea that's how we should live.

This is why a lot of the exercises on these pages are about plotting the future and having a think about who we are, so that we can better see a plausible and enjoyable way forward that is appropriate for us. And when we can see a way forward, it is more enjoyable and healthier if we can then break it down into bite-sized chunks.

Have a little think now to see if some of the above kind of thinking is what motivated you to buy this book. If so then at the end, or tomorrow when you pick it up again, you will want to look through the pages highlighting the strategies that help you to:

1 Improve the quality of your present day life.

2 Enjoy what you already have more.

3 Understand better who you are and what would be reasonable paths for your future.

4 Break this down into do-able chunks.

You may want to start now, by looking at your list of traits and your list of five things you want to do in the next year. You may now want to get a fresh piece of paper and choose two or three broader goals for the year after that. It might be a trip, it might be a career change, it might be starting a new business, it might be enrolling for a course, it might be improving the work you already do.

Now, for argument's sake, pick the most attainable of these. Write this goal at the bottom of a piece of paper. Write the word 'Now' at the top of the page. Now write some little bite size do-able tasks between the two that will slowly make this happen. You may even want to put some rough dates beside these items. For instance, say you wanted to train for a better or different job: you would put the name of the job at the bottom, then perhaps the course you have to go on in the middle of the page, and then perhaps above that you would put how you will go about finding the money for the course. Perhaps you will also add how you will find the time for the course and any practical issues like finding childcare if you are a parent, or accommodation if would need to move, or the time if you are working. You might want to write some of the solutions to these problems on the right hand side of the sheet.

Does your goal now look do-able? If not, try the exercise with another goal you might like to achieve in the next couple of years. The first choice goal might be for a few year's time perhaps.

Leave your sheet in plain view.

We are getting to the end of our notional session, so we need to reinforce a few positive techniques and make sure they are lodged firmly in our brains.

Firstly go back to the 'mirror' exercise in chapter 7 and repeat the exercise for one of your problems: probably the first problem you chose. Watch your lips in the mirror as you enunciate the problem. Then put the mirror down and visualise the problem on a blank piece of paper. Then reduce it and drain it of motion and colour. Then crumple it up and put it in the bin.

Now:

Sit up straight.

Clap your hands twice.

Clap your hands twice more.

Say out loud,

NO **ONE** CURE WILL CHANGE MY LIFE 100%.

Now smile and twinkle your eyes. Keep smiling and twinkling while you say out loud,

SEN-SAY-SHUN-AL.

SHINING.

FAN-TAST-TIC.

GOR-GEOUS.

FA-BU-LOUS.

HAPPY.

HIL-AIR-IOUS.

SEN-SUAL.

GLITTERING.

I CAN DO ANYTHING.

I CAN DO ANYTHING.

I CAN DO ANYTHING.

Now look in the bin and take out the pieces of paper that are in there.

Unfurl them and look long and hard at what's on them.

How do you feel at this moment?

THE LIST OF THINGS TO DO (from chapter nine): if you have read this book in the evening, then tomorrow is your crux day for this. You must address the tasks you have set out. If you do this, a huge burden will disappear. You will feel energised and dynamic and you will feel you have seized control of your life and that everything now becomes possible. If you get to tomorrow and you chicken out and wilt, then this is because you have *decided* not to move forward. After all, you chose the problems on the list and you have clearly written what you *can* do to solve them. It is up to you. You know how fabulous you will feel when you carry out the solutions you have listed. You will feel FAN-TA-STIC. Go for it.

To recap what we have learnt today:

Depression is an illness that tries to rob you of the very skills and energies you need to fight it.

No one measure will change your life 100%, you need to look for fifty or more small changes, and actually carry them out.

Get more exercise.

Examine the interests you already have and have had in the past. Diversify them and add to them. It may be helpful to come up with some bite-sized targets.

Improve your relationships by giving more back and respecting people for who they are. If all things are even in a relationship, be a big person, not a whiner.

Regularly use the exercises listed in this book. Visualisations, breathing exercises, exercises before you go to sleep. You will then feel SEN-SAY-SHUN-ALL.

Make realistic plans for the future and carry them out. Life is for living. Get out there and live it.

Learn and explore new skills which will help your brain like self-hypnosis, cognitive therapy, and items from the list coming up.

Don't see everything as a battle or a threat to your status. What would someone you admire do?

Eat better, cut down on the booze.

Never ever say or think, 'Oh I can't be bothered.'

Learn to love your own company.

Review your week and look to increase the 'little' treats in life.

Ignore the phoney dreams we get through the media, or the fake needs like wanting to be in with the smart set. Read your sheet of positive traits. This is who you are. Be proud of it. Play to your strengths in your daily life.

Don't look for other people to solve your problems for you. Why on earth would it be their job?

Now choose some more things to do and fill your days ahead with them. The total number of tasks should take you over the 'fifty' mark...

1   Take up Kick Boxing.

2   Try 'writing out.' Turn the lights low – maybe light a candle and sit in front of a computer or get a pad of paper and write and write and write. Just follow your stream of thoughts. Don't read what you have written. Just keep writing and never read what you have written so far and don't worry about grammar, spelling or punctuation. After 20 minutes of this you will feel as though you have given your brain a good clear out.

3   Try to throw yourself into your work for a whole week. Enjoy doing everything that little bit better and let it be your own little secret; don't look for recognition.

4   Bach Flower essences.

5   Take a dog for a walk. You may have to borrow a dog. Many vets also welcome volunteer dog walkers.

6   Force yourself to act normal. Your brain is telling you not to do stuff; it's even telling you not to have fun. Make yourself do that fun thing, regardless of what your brain tells you.

7   Spend more time listening to *other* people's problems. If someone looks down in the mouth. Ask them if you can help or if they want to talk.

8   Read something frivolous; P.G. Wodehouse books or something aimed at youngsters.

9   Take some small part of your environment, like a cupboard, drawer, sink or the glove compartment of your car, and clean it out. It will show you that you really can be effective.

10 Move around during the day as much as possible. People who are below the average UK weight spend an average of two hours a day extra on their feet compared to people over the average weight.

11 Keep your spine erect. Do not slump when sitting or standing. Posture can have a tremendous, quick effect on mood.

12 Become more aware of how other people make you feel. Learn to mentally dismiss people who leave you feeling lower.

13 Have a big clearout and send all the clutter off to either the local charity shop or the tip, depending on its condition.

14 Smile at strangers. Smile more at people you know.

15 If you hate being on your own, leave a movie on the TV that you already know well. Perhaps tapes of a sitcom you like.

16 Get a fish tank. They are absorbing to gaze at and offer lots of little jobs to do.

17 Learn three jokes. There are lots of websites such as FHM.com that have them or ask a few people what their all time favourite joke is. Here's one to start you off.

Q: Why did the spirit cross the road?

A: To get to the other side.

I didn't say it was *good* joke.

18 Volunteer to do hospital visiting.

19 Take up drawing and painting.

20 Listen to books on tape while driving to and from work (instead of the same old music or bad news on the radio) it helps to stimulate the mind and distracts from problems.

21 Yoga.

22 Raw Broccoli. Broccoli is packed with B vitamins, anti-oxidants, anti-cancer chemicals. It keeps you alert and eases the stresses of life. Apparently.

23 Keep lists, like the one we did earlier – 'five things I want to achieve' – 'five bands I want to see' 'five teams I want to see' 'five places I want to go to.' When you look at the list years later you will be amazed at how many you have achieved.

24 Visualize/give a name to/ somehow characterize your depression.

It will help you recognize it when it strikes- then you can just say, 'Oh, that's just Jerry or My Bag of Slimy Rocks or my Gremlin'. And also respect its power. By that I mean, don't be scared of it, but respect the danger it poses to you, so that you can avoid it. We can't detonate all our mental/emotional land mines but we can clearly mark them and stay away.

25 Meditation.

26 Get in your car and go for an exhilarating drive. It doesn't matter where.

27 Give yourself little treats after completing a task that you don't like.

28 Think more in terms of progress and less in terms of perfection.

29 Become your own best friend.

30 You would do practically anything for a best friend. So why don't we always do the same for our partner?

31 Stay busy.

32 Take chances – within reason.

33 Do one extra act of kindness every day.

34 Don't sit if you can stand. Don't stand if you can walk. Don't use transport if you can walk. Don't walk, if you can jog.

35 Try something you have never tried before, no matter how small.

36 Don't belittle the little pleasures: they are the stuff of life.

37 Find something or someone to nurture: it is often one of the elements missing from modern life.

38 Take ten extra minutes out in the sunshine when you can.

39 Cultivate a secret passion and read up on it. Orchids, a favourite artist, history...

40 Join an evening class to learn or improve the next language you will need, either for your next holiday or to help with customers. Get a CD of that language and leave it on 'repeat' as you get on with your life around the house or as you drive. It's astonishing how much will go into your brain and stay there.

41 When we are depressed we frequently stop looking after ourselves so well. We might not dress so well, or we might let our living environment get more untidy and dirty. Conversely we think of well dressed people

who are smart and live in a smart house as being mentally well. Interestingly therefore, it has been shown that when we smarten ourselves up and when we clean and tidy the house, we associate the act with feeling good: feeling well and dynamic. So... do a little job you've been putting off, like giving the bathroom a really good clean, or cleaning under the bed. Get a clock, and before starting, time yourself so that you are sure you worked for, say, a genuine half an hour before having a break.

42 Look at the time. Absolutely forbid yourself to think anything negative for one whole hour. After the hour give yourself a little treat. You managed it for one hour. Why not do it for the rest of the day?

43 Re-write the past. If you have an episode from the past that made you anxious, start writing about it using a good paragraph of recognisable details and then continue writing but now adding differences: a story where things turn out better or funnier or happier. Why not add a space alien or three? They could kidnap someone you hated. It doesn't matter how silly it all gets.

44 Accept all social invitations. If you don't know anyone at a party, look for someone who also looks 'left out of it' and introduce yourself by saying 'I don't know anyone here: my name is...' they may be lonely and you will make their day. They could turn out to be your new best friend or a complete waste of space: you won't know until you say hello.

45 Baby-sit for a friend who needs to get out.

46 Sit down with your finances and follow that good advice we all hear but ignore. For example, move to a credit card with a 0% deal then move to another one when that deal expires. For the fun or it, ring your mortgage company or mobile phone supplier and say you are thinking of leaving and going for a better deal elsewhere. See what they offer you.

47 Spot something in your routine that makes your heart sink but which is necessary, and act as if you like it. For example, get to work ten minutes early.

48 Successful people tend to be interested in other successful people. For example, when we are feeling good about ourselves, we are more likely to want to read a book about someone like Richard Branson. Choose a book about someone successful and read it: it will make you feel much more positive and 'can do.'

49 It is NOT someone else's job to make us happy. Only you can do it for yourself. I know I have said this before. It is crucial to understand it.

50 Don't dwell on life. Live it.

Go back through this book highlighting or bookmarking the exercises and ideas you would like to prioritise for the next few days. Go back through this book looking for bits you didn't bother with the first time. Go back through this book and earmark exercises you will need to do a) every day b) last thing at night, and c) when you need a 'boost' or feel anxieties. In a few weeks or months you may have issues that are bugging you that aren't identical to the ones you have explored today. Get this book back off your bookshelf and do some of the exercises with these new concerns in mind; it will reinforce the good work you've done today, and help to tidy up different, more peripheral issues in your life.

Finally:

Sit up straight. Smile. Twinkle your eyes. How do you feel?

SEN-SAY-SHUN-AL.

About the author

Paul Vincent has made numerous appearances on radio and television discussing various aspects of mental health and how we can all learn to enjoy our lives more. He has also worked for Radio 4 and is the author of bestselling thrillers and comedies including: *The Textbook Man, Free, The Death of Me* and *Meet The Hormones.*

Printed in the United Kingdom
by Lightning Source UK Ltd.
125418UK00001B/29/A